Quick and easy complete solution Crohn's disease diet cookbook: for seniors

Enjoy the complete delicious recipes to balance and cure your healthy, + seniors 28day meal plan to stay Longlife.

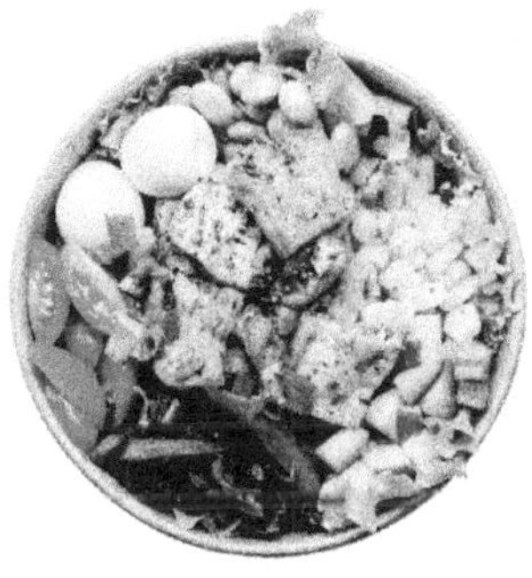

Dr. Jerry Cole

TABLE OF CONTENT

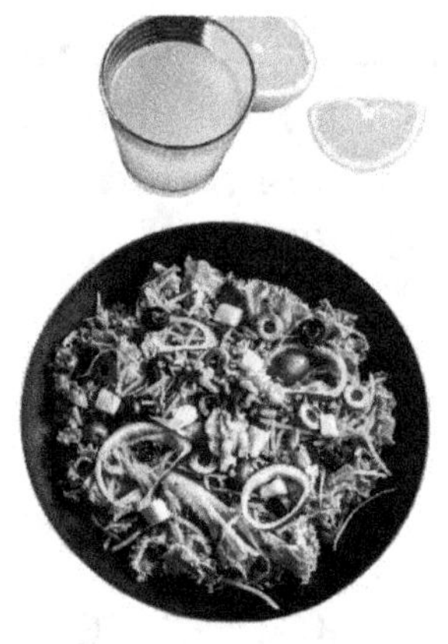

INTRODUCTION

"Living with Crohn's disease as a senior can be especially challenging. Managing symptoms, navigating dietary restrictions, and finding the energy to cook can feel overwhelming. But with the right tools and support, you can take control of your health and enjoy delicious, nutritious meals that soothe your symptoms and nourish your body.

This Quick and Easy Complete Solution Crohn's Disease Diet Cookbook for Seniors is designed specifically with your needs in mind. With easy-to-follow recipes, simple ingredient lists, and gentle cooking methods, you'll be able to prepare healthy, Crohn's-friendly meals in no time. From comforting breakfasts to satisfying dinners, and even sweet treats, this cookbook has everything you need to thrive with Crohn's disease.

In this cookbook, we'll show you how to:

- Identify and avoid trigger foods
- Incorporate gut-healing ingredients
- Make cooking and meal prep a breeze
- Enjoy flavorful, nutritious meals that support your health

Take the first step towards a happier, healthier you. Let this cookbook be your guide on the journey to managing your Crohn's disease and living your best life."

- Acknowledge the unique challenges of living with Crohn's disease as a senior
- Offer a solution that addresses these challenges
- Highlight the benefits of the cookbook, including easy-to-follow recipes and gentle cooking methods
- Encourage the reader to take control of their health and thrive with Crohn's disease.

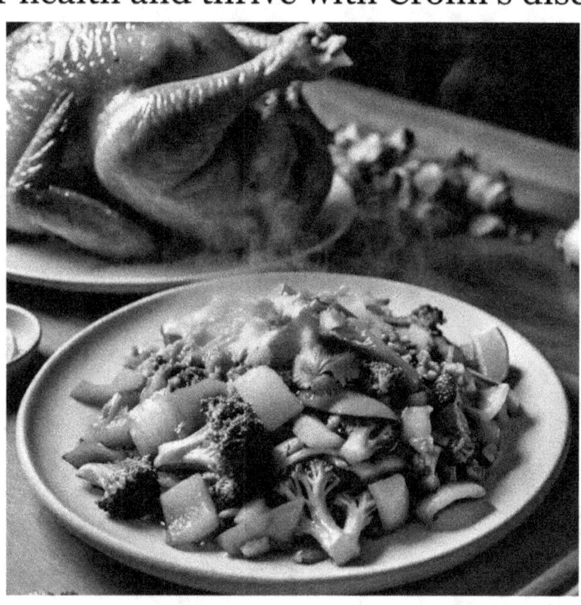

DESCRIBE CROHN'S DISEASE

A chronic inflammatory disease mostly affecting the gastrointestinal (GI) tract is called Crohn's disease. Like ulcerative colitis, it is categorized as an inflammatory bowel disease (IBD). Although Crohn's disease can affect any area of the gastrointestinal tract, including the mouth and the anus, it most frequently affects the small intestine and the colon, which is the start of the large intestine.

Although the precise origin of Crohn's disease is unknown, a combination of immunological abnormality, environmental factors, and genetic predisposition is thought to be responsible. Crohn's disease symptoms can differ greatly from person to person and can include fever, exhaustion, diarrhea, weight loss, and rectal bleeding.

Usually, a mix of drugs is used to inhibit the immune system, regulate inflammation, and manage symptoms. Surgery could be required in some circumstances to cure complications like strictures or fistulas or to remove damaged sections of the gut. Although Crohn's disease is a chronic illness that needs to be managed continuously, many patients with the disease can have active, fulfilling lives if they receive the right care.

SENIORS' PAIN RELIEF CROHN'S DISEASE

Seniors with Crohn's disease require a multimodal approach to pain management, which may include prescription drugs, lifestyle modifications, and complementary therapies. Here are a few tactics that are often employed:

Medication: Because NSAIDs have the potential to exacerbate symptoms, it is typically advised to avoid them when treating Crohn's disease. Alternatively, low-dose opioids recommended by a medical practitioner or drugs like acetaminophen (Tylenol) may be used to relieve pain. Furthermore, pain may be indirectly reduced by drugs used to manage Crohn's disease symptoms and reduce inflammation.

Dietary adjustments: Depending on their specific requirements and dietary tolerances, seniors with Crohn's disease may benefit from dietary adjustments. Pain and discomfort may be lessened by avoiding trigger foods that intensify symptoms, such as spicy or high-fiber foods, and by concentrating on a well-balanced diet full of easily digested foods.

Stress management: Stress can increase pain and aggravate Crohn's disease symptoms. Stress-reduction strategies for seniors, such as deep breathing, relaxation training, meditation, and fun hobbies, can be beneficial.

Physical activity: Engaging in regular physical activity can enhance general wellbeing and potentially reduce Crohn's disease symptoms, such as discomfort. Seniors should exercise according to their fitness level, such as swimming, walking, or light yoga, under the supervision of a healthcare professional.

Complementary therapies: Acupuncture, massage therapy, and hypnosis are examples of complementary therapies that some seniors use to relieve pain. These therapies ought to be administered under the supervision of a licensed healthcare provider and in addition to standard medical treatments.

Supportive care: To help seniors with Crohn's disease deal with the psychological effects of having a chronic illness, support groups or counseling may be beneficial. Developing a relationship with people who can relate to their experiences can be a great way to get support and motivation.

Seniors with Crohn's disease should collaborate closely with their medical professionals to create a customized pain management strategy that meets their unique requirements and preferences. For the best possible pain relief and overall quality of life, treatment plan modifications and routine monitoring may be required.

SENIORS: BEGINNING THE PROCESS CROHN'S DISEASE

Seniors who have Crohn's disease must take some important actions to begin managing the condition:

Consultation with a healthcare professional: To discuss their symptoms and receive a full evaluation, seniors should make an appointment with a gastroenterologist, a physician who specializes in digestive disorders. In order to confirm the diagnosis and determine the severity of the illness, the gastroenterologist will probably conduct a physical examination, go over the patient's medical history, and request testing such blood or stool tests, imaging investigations, or endoscopic procedures.

Creation of a treatment plan: The healthcare professional will collaborate with the senior to create a thorough treatment plan that is suited to their specific needs based on the evaluation results. Medication to manage symptoms, reduce inflammation, and weaken the immune system may be part of this strategy. It might also be advised to make dietary adjustments, lifestyle adjustments, or use complementary therapies.

Education and self-care: Seniors have a responsibility to actively learn about Crohn's disease, including symptoms, causes, available treatments, and possible side effects. Healthcare professionals can offer elders support and educational materials to help them better understand their health and learn how to take care of themselves. This could entail following prescription schedules, recognizing and treating flare-ups, and adjusting one's food and way of life.

Dietary adjustments: Depending on their specific requirements and dietary tolerances, seniors with Crohn's disease may benefit from dietary adjustments. Seniors can identify trigger foods and create a well-balanced diet that supports their general health and manages their symptoms by working with a trained dietitian or nutritionist.

Frequent monitoring and follow-up: In order to evaluate their response to treatment, keep an eye out for any complications, and modify the treatment plan as necessary, seniors with Crohn's disease need regular monitoring and follow-up care. Regular check-ups, tests, and consultations will be scheduled by healthcare specialists to guarantee that the senior's condition is adequately handled.

Supportive care: Managing the physical and psychological effects of Crohn's disease can be difficult for seniors. They may find it helpful to attend support groups, seek therapy, or get other forms of emotional support. Making connections with people who have similar experiences to them can be a great way to get helpful guidance, support, and encouragement.

Seniors who manage their Crohn's disease pro-actively, in close collaboration with healthcare professionals, can limit complications, efficiently manage symptoms, and enhance their quality of life.

CROHN'S DISEASE COOKING WITH THE ELDERLY

In order to manage symptoms and support general health, cooking for seniors with Crohn's disease necessitates careful consideration of their dietary preferences and sensitivities. The following advice can help elders with Crohn's disease while they cook:

Low-Fiber Diet: For many elderly Crohn's disease patients, a low-fiber diet helps manage symptoms including diarrhea and stomach pain. In general, digestibility is facilitated by cooked or peeled fruits and vegetables, refined grains, and thoroughly cooked meats. Steer clear of high-fiber foods such as tough cuts of meat, whole grains, nuts, seeds, and fresh fruits and vegetables.

Small, Regular Meals: Rather than consuming large meals throughout the day, seniors with Crohn's disease may discover that eating smaller, more often meals is beneficial. By doing so, symptoms like bloating and pain can be reduced and the digestive system's risk of overloading is reduced.

Avoid Food Triggers: Some foods have the potential to cause flare-ups in the symptoms of Crohn's disease. Caffeine, alcohol, dairy products, and fatty foods are common triggers. When organizing meals, keep note of which foods aggravate your symptoms and steer clear of them.

Cooking Techniques: Opt for cooking techniques like steaming, boiling, baking, or grilling that are easy on the digestive system. Steer clear of frying and heavy oil use because fatty foods might aggravate symptoms.

Hydration: Due to diarrhea and fluid loss, seniors with Crohn's disease are more likely to get dehydrated. Offer water, herbal teas, clear broths, and electrolyte-rich drinks, such as coconut water, throughout the day to promote proper hydration.

Foods High in Protein: Including foods high in protein in meals can assist seniors maintain their energy levels and muscle strength. Choose lean protein sources including fish, eggs, tofu, chicken, and lentils. Pay attention to portion amounts and stay away from fatty or highly processed meats.

Nutrient-Dense items: To enhance general health and wellness, concentrate on adding nutrient-dense items to meals. Leafy greens, vibrant fruits and vegetables, whole grains (if acceptable), nuts, seeds, avocado, and olive oil are a few examples of good fats.

Food Safety: Because seniors with Crohn's disease may have compromised immune systems, it's critical to put food safety first while preparing meals. Aim to prevent cross-contamination between raw and cooked foods, cook food to the proper temperature, and thoroughly wash hands, utensils, and surfaces.

Think About Food Supplements: To make sure they're getting the nutrients they need, seniors with Crohn's disease may occasionally benefit from taking nutritional supplements. Consult a dietician or healthcare professional to find out if taking probiotics, vitamin B12, or D supplements can help.

Promote Pleasurable Meals: Seniors should, whenever feasible, be involved in the planning and preparation of their meals since eating should be a joyful experience. Embrace their dietary constraints while incorporating their favorite flavors and foods into meals.

You may support seniors with Crohn's disease nutritionally, control their symptoms, and enhance their general wellbeing by cooking with these considerations in mind.

DAY 1:

Breakfast: Oatmeal with mashed banana and a sprinkle of ground flaxseeds.

Lunch: Grilled chicken breast with steamed carrots and mashed sweet potatoes.

Snack: Rice cakes with almond butter.

Dinner: Baked salmon with quinoa and steamed spinach.

Day 2:

Breakfast: Smoothie made with lactose-free yogurt, spinach, frozen berries, and a scoop of protein powder.

Lunch: Turkey and avocado wrap with lettuce and gluten-free tortilla.

Snack: Greek yogurt with honey and a handful of walnuts.

Dinner: Stir-fried tofu with bell peppers and brown rice.

Day 3:

Breakfast: Scrambled eggs with sautéed spinach and gluten-free toast.

Lunch: Lentil soup with a side of gluten-free crackers.

Snack: Apple slices with peanut butter.

Dinner: Baked cod with roasted asparagus and quinoa.

Day 4:

Breakfast: Quinoa porridge with cinnamon, diced pear, and a drizzle of maple syrup.

Lunch: Chicken and vegetable stir-fry with rice noodles.

Snack: Cottage cheese with pineapple chunks.

Dinner: Turkey meatballs with zucchini noodles and marinara sauce.

Day 5:

Breakfast: Smoothie bowl topped with sliced banana, chia seeds, and granola.

Lunch: Spinach salad with grilled shrimp, cherry tomatoes, and balsamic vinaigrette.

Snack: Rice pudding made with coconut milk and a sprinkle of cinnamon.

Dinner: Baked chicken thighs with roasted Brussels sprouts and quinoa.

Day 6:

Breakfast: Buckwheat pancakes topped with Greek yogurt and mixed berries.

Lunch: Quinoa salad with chickpeas, cucumber, tomato, and lemon-tahini dressing.

Snack: Celery sticks with hummus.

Dinner: Baked trout with steamed green beans and mashed cauliflower.

Day 7:

Breakfast: Chia seed pudding made with almond milk and topped with sliced mango and shredded coconut.

Lunch: Turkey and avocado salad with mixed greens, cucumber, and balsamic vinaigrette.

Snack: Rice cakes with mashed avocado and tomato slices.

Dinner: Beef stew with carrots, potatoes, and served over mashed sweet potatoes.

Day 8

Breakfast: Smoothie made with lactose-free yogurt, banana, spinach, and a tablespoon of almond butter.

Lunch: Grilled salmon salad with mixed greens, cherry tomatoes, and a light vinaigrette dressing.

Snack: Rice crackers with tuna salad (made with canned tuna, mayo, and diced celery).

Dinner: Baked chicken breast with steamed broccoli and quinoa.

Day 9:

Breakfast: Scrambled eggs with sautéed bell peppers, mushrooms, and gluten-free toast.

Lunch: Turkey and vegetable stir-fry with rice noodles.

Snack: Cottage cheese with sliced peaches.

Dinner: Baked cod with roasted Brussels sprouts and mashed sweet potatoes.

Day 10:

Breakfast: Oatmeal with mashed raspberries and a sprinkle of chia seeds.
Lunch: Lentil soup with gluten-free crackers.
Snack: Apple slices with almond butter.
Dinner: Grilled chicken thighs with steamed carrots and brown rice.

Day 11:

Breakfast: Smoothie bowl topped with kiwi slices, shredded coconut, and a drizzle of honey.
Lunch: Spinach salad with grilled shrimp, avocado, and a citrus vinaigrette.
Snack: Rice cakes with hummus and cucumber slices.
Dinner: Turkey meatballs with marinara sauce over zucchini noodles.

Day 12:

Breakfast: Buckwheat pancakes with sliced strawberries and a dollop of Greek yogurt.
Lunch: Quinoa salad with chickpeas, cucumber, tomato, and lemon-tahini dressing.
Snack: Celery sticks with almond butter.
Dinner: Baked trout with roasted asparagus and mashed cauliflower.

Day 13:

Breakfast: Chia seed pudding made with coconut milk, topped with mango chunks and a sprinkle of granola.
Lunch: Chicken and vegetable wrap with lettuce, tomato, and gluten-free tortilla.
Snack: Greek yogurt with honey and a handful of walnuts.

Dinner: Beef stew with carrots, potatoes, and served over mashed potatoes.

Day 14:

Breakfast: Smoothie made with spinach, banana, frozen berries, and a scoop of protein powder.
Lunch: Tuna salad stuffed in a bell pepper with a side of carrot sticks.
Snack: Rice crackers with guacamole.
Dinner: Grilled salmon with quinoa pilaf and steamed green beans.

Day 15:

Breakfast: Overnight oats made with almond milk, topped with sliced banana and a sprinkle of cinnamon.
Lunch: Turkey and avocado wrap with lettuce and gluten-free tortilla.

Snack: Rice cakes with hummus and cucumber slices.
Dinner: Baked chicken breast with steamed carrots and quinoa.

Day 16:

Breakfast: Smoothie bowl topped with mixed berries, shredded coconut, and a drizzle of honey.
Lunch: Lentil soup with gluten-free crackers.
Snack: Greek yogurt with sliced peaches and a handful of almonds.
Dinner: Grilled salmon with roasted Brussels sprouts and mashed sweet potatoes.

Day 17:

Breakfast: Scrambled eggs with sautéed spinach and gluten-free toast.

Lunch: Chicken and vegetable stir-fry with rice noodles.
Snack: Apple slices with almond butter.
Dinner: Baked cod with quinoa pilaf and steamed asparagus.

Day 18:

Breakfast: Buckwheat pancakes with sliced strawberries and a dollop of lactose-free yogurt.
Lunch: Spinach salad with grilled shrimp, avocado, and a light vinaigrette dressing.
Snack: Rice crackers with tuna salad (made with canned tuna, mayo, and diced celery).
Dinner: Turkey meatballs with marinara sauce over zucchini noodles.

Day 19:

Breakfast: Chia seed pudding made with coconut milk, topped with mango chunks and a sprinkle of granola.
Lunch: Quinoa salad with chickpeas, cucumber, tomato, and lemon-tahini dressing.
Snack: Cottage cheese with pineapple chunks.
Dinner: Baked trout with roasted asparagus and mashed cauliflower.

Day 20:

Breakfast: Smoothie made with spinach, banana, frozen berries, and a scoop of protein powder.
Lunch: Tuna salad stuffed in a bell pepper with a side of carrot sticks.
Snack: Rice cakes with mashed avocado and tomato slices.
Dinner: Beef stew with carrots, potatoes, and served over mashed potatoes.

Day 21:

Breakfast: Oatmeal with mashed raspberries and a sprinkle of chia seeds.
Lunch: Grilled chicken thighs with steamed green beans and brown rice.
Snack: Celery sticks with hummus.
Dinner: Baked salmon with quinoa and steamed broccoli.

Day 22:

Breakfast: Smoothie made with lactose-free yogurt, spinach, frozen berries, and a tablespoon of almond butter.
Lunch: Turkey and avocado wrap with lettuce and gluten-free tortilla.
Snack: Rice cakes with hummus and cucumber slices.
Dinner: Baked chicken breast with steamed carrots and quinoa.

Day 23:

Breakfast: Oatmeal with mashed banana and a sprinkle of ground flaxseeds.
Lunch: Lentil soup with gluten-free crackers.
Snack: Greek yogurt with sliced peaches and a handful of almonds.
Dinner: Grilled salmon with roasted Brussels sprouts and mashed sweet potatoes.

Day 24:

Breakfast: Scrambled eggs with sautéed spinach and gluten-free toast.
Lunch: Chicken and vegetable stir-fry with rice noodles.
Snack: Apple slices with almond butter.
Dinner: Baked cod with quinoa pilaf and steamed asparagus.

Day 25:

Breakfast: Smoothie bowl topped with mixed berries, shredded coconut, and a drizzle of honey.
Lunch: Spinach salad with grilled shrimp, avocado, and a light vinaigrette dressing.
Snack: Rice crackers with tuna salad (made with canned tuna, mayo, and diced celery).
Dinner: Turkey meatballs with marinara sauce over zucchini noodles.

Day 26:

Breakfast: Chia seed pudding made with coconut milk, topped with mango chunks and a sprinkle of granola.
Lunch: Quinoa salad with chickpeas, cucumber, tomato, and lemon-tahini dressing.

Snack: Cottage cheese with pineapple chunks.

Dinner: Baked trout with roasted asparagus and mashed cauliflower.

Breakfast: Smoothie made with spinach, banana, frozen berries, and a scoop of protein powder.

Lunch: Tuna salad stuffed in a bell pepper with a side of carrot sticks.

Snack: Rice cakes with mashed avocado and tomato slices.

Dinner: Beef stew with carrots, potatoes, and served over mashed potatoes.

Breakfast: Oatmeal with mashed raspberries and a sprinkle of chia seeds.

Lunch: Grilled chicken thighs with steamed green beans and brown rice.

Snack: Celery sticks with hummus.

Dinner: Baked salmon with quinoa and steamed broccoli.

BREAKFAST RECIPES

Banana Oatmeal Smoothie

Ingredients:

- 1 cup rolled oats
- 1 banana
- 1 cup milk (dairy or non-dairy)
- 1/2 cup plain Greek yogurt
- 1 tablespoon honey (optional)
- 1/2 teaspoon ground cinnamon

Instructions:

1. In a blender, combine the oats, banana, milk, yogurt, honey (if using), and cinnamon.
2. Blend until smooth and creamy.

3. Adjust consistency by adding more milk if too thick or ice cubes if too thin.
4. Pour into a glass and enjoy.

Avocado Toast with Scrambled Eggs

Ingredients:

- 2 slices whole-grain bread
- 1 ripe avocado
- 2 eggs
- 1 tablespoon milk or water
- Salt and pepper to taste

Instructions

1. Toast the bread slices.
2. Mash the avocado and spread it evenly on the toasted bread.
3. In a small bowl, whisk the eggs with milk or water and a pinch of salt and pepper.
4. Cook the scrambled eggs in a non-stick pan over medium heat, stirring occasionally.

5. Top the avocado toast with the scrambled eggs.

Quinoa Porridge with Berries

Ingredients:
- 1 cup cooked quinoa
- 1 cup milk (dairy or non-dairy)
- 1/2 cup mixed berries (e.g., strawberries, blueberries, raspberries)
- 1 tablespoon honey or maple syrup
- 1/4 teaspoon ground cinnamon

Instructions
1. In a saucepan, combine the cooked quinoa and milk.
2. Heat the mixture over medium-low heat, stirring occasionally, until it reaches the desired consistency.
3. Remove from heat and stir in the berries, honey or maple syrup, and cinnamon.
4. Serve warm.

Greek Yogurt Parfait

Ingredients:

- 1 cup plain Greek yogurt
- 1/2 cup granola (look for low-fiber options)
- 1/2 cup fresh or frozen fruit (e.g., berries, peaches, mango)
- 1 tablespoon honey or maple syrup (optional)

Instructions

1. In a parfait glass or bowl, layer half of the yogurt, followed by half of the granola and half of the fruit.
2. Repeat the layers with the remaining yogurt, granola, and fruit.
3. Drizzle with honey or maple syrup, if desired.

Egg Muffin Cups

Ingredients:

- 6 eggs
- 1/4 cup milk or water
- 1/2 cup diced cooked vegetables (e.g., spinach, bell peppers, onions)
- Salt and pepper to taste

Instructions

1. Preheat the oven to 350°F (175°C).
2. Grease a muffin tin or use silicone muffin cups.
3. In a bowl, whisk together the eggs and milk or water. Season with salt and pepper.
4. Divide the diced vegetables evenly among the muffin cups.
5. Pour the egg mixture over the vegetables, filling the cups about 3/4 full.
6. Bake for 15-20 minutes, or until the eggs are set.
7. Remove from the oven and let cool slightly before serving.

LUNCH RECIPES

Baked Sweet Potato with Tuna Salad

Ingredients:

- 2 medium sweet potatoes
- 1 (5 oz) can tuna, drained
- 1/4 cup plain Greek yogurt

- 2 tablespoons diced celery
- 2 tablespoons diced red onion
- 1 tablespoon lemon juice
- Salt and pepper to taste

Instructions

1. Preheat the oven to 400°F (200°C).
2. Wash the sweet potatoes and prick them with a fork.
3. Bake the sweet potatoes for 45-60 minutes, or until tender when pierced with a fork.
4. In a bowl, combine the drained tuna, Greek yogurt, celery, red onion, lemon juice, and salt and pepper to taste.
5. Cut the baked sweet potatoes lengthwise and top with the tuna salad.

Quinoa and Vegetable Soup

Ingredients:

- 1 cup cooked quinoa
- 4 cups low-sodium vegetable or chicken broth
- 1 cup diced carrots

- 1 cup diced zucchini
- 1/2 cup diced celery
- Salt and pepper to taste
- Fresh herbs (e.g., parsley, dill) for garnish (option)

Instructions

1. In a saucepan, bring the broth to a boil.
2. Add the carrots, zucchini, and celery. Reduce heat to medium-low and simmer for 10-15 minutes, or until the vegetables are tender.
3. Stir in the cooked quinoa and season with salt and pepper to taste.
4. Garnish with fresh herbs if desired.

Egg Salad Lettuce Wraps

Ingredients:
- 4 hard-boiled eggs, chopped
- 1/4 cup plain Greek yogurt
- 2 tablespoons diced celery
- 2 tablespoons diced red onion
- 1 tablespoon Dijon mustard
- Salt and pepper to taste

- Lettuce leaves (e.g., romaine, butter lettuce) for wrapping

Instructions

1. In a bowl, combine the chopped hard-boiled eggs, Greek yogurt, celery, red onion, Dijon mustard, and salt and pepper to taste.
2. Spoon the egg salad mixture into lettuce leaves and wrap them up.

Grilled Chicken Salad

Ingredients:

- 4 oz grilled chicken breast, sliced
- 2 cups mixed greens or baby spinach
- 1/2 cup sliced cucumber
- 1/4 cup sliced red bell pepper
- 2 tablespoons olive oil
- 2 tablespoons lemon juice or vinegar
- Salt and pepper to taste

Instructions

1. In a large bowl, combine the mixed greens or baby spinach, sliced cucumber, and sliced red bell pepper.

2. In a small bowl, whisk together the olive oil, lemon juice or vinegar, and salt and pepper to make a simple dressing.

3. Add the sliced grilled chicken to the salad and drizzle with the dressing.

Hummus and Vegetable Wrap

Ingredients:

- 1 whole wheat tortilla or wrap
- 1/4 cup hummus
- 1/2 cup sliced cucumbers
- 1/4 cup sliced red bell pepper
- 1/4 cup shredded carrots

Instructions

1. Spread the hummus evenly over the tortilla or wrap.

2. Layer the sliced cucumbers, red bell pepper, and shredded carrots on one side of the tortilla or wrap.

3. Carefully roll up the tortilla or wrap, tucking in the sides as you go.

4. Slice in half and serve.

Baked Salmon with Roasted Vegetables

Ingredients:

- 4 (4 oz) salmon fillets
- 2 cups diced potatoes
- 1 cup diced carrots
- 1 cup diced zucchini
- 2 tablespoons olive oil
- Salt and pepper to taste
- Lemon wedges for serving

Instructions

1. Preheat the oven to 400°F (200°C).
2. In a large bowl, toss the diced potatoes, carrots, and zucchini with olive oil, salt, and pepper.
3. Spread the vegetable mixture on a baking sheet.
4. Place the salmon fillets on the same baking sheet, or on a separate sheet if preferred.

5. Bake for 20-25 minutes, or until the salmon is cooked through and the vegetables are tender.
6. Serve the salmon and roasted vegetables with lemon wedges.

Lentil and Sweet Potato Curry

Ingredients:
- 1 cup dried lentils, rinsed
- 1 medium sweet potato, peeled and diced
- 1 (14 oz) can diced tomatoes
- 1 cup vegetable or chicken broth
- 1 tablespoon curry powder
- 1 teaspoon ground cumin
- Salt and pepper to taste
- Fresh cilantro for garnish (optional)

Instructions
1. In a large saucepan, combine the lentils, sweet potato, diced tomatoes, broth, curry powder, cumin, salt, and pepper.
2. Bring the mixture to a boil, then reduce heat to low, cover, and simmer

for 20-25 minutes, or until the lentils and sweet potato are tender.

3. Adjust the consistency by adding more broth if needed.

4. Garnish with fresh cilantro if desired.

Turkey Meatballs with Zucchini Noodles

Ingredients:

- 1 lb ground turkey
- 1 egg
- 1/4 cup breadcrumbs
- 1/4 cup grated Parmesan cheese
- 1 teaspoon dried basil
- 1 teaspoon dried oregano
- Salt and pepper to taste
- 2 medium zucchini, spiralized or julienned
- 1 cup marinara sauce

Instructions

1. Preheat the oven to 400°F (200°C).

2. In a bowl, combine the ground turkey, egg, breadcrumbs, Parmesan cheese, basil, oregano, salt, and pepper. Mix well and form into meatballs.

3. Place the meatballs on a baking sheet and bake for 15-20 minutes, or until cooked through.
4. While the meatballs are baking, prepare the zucchini noodles by spiralizing or julienning the zucchini.
5. In a skillet, heat the marinara sauce and add the zucchini noodles. Cook for 2-3 minutes, or until the noodles are slightly softened.
6. Serve the turkey meatballs over the zucchini noodles with marinara sauce.

Chicken and Rice Casserole

Ingredients:
- 2 cups cooked and shredded chicken
- 1 cup cooked brown rice
- 1 (10.5 oz) can condensed cream of mushroom soup
- 1/2 cup milk
- 1 cup frozen mixed vegetables
- 1/4 cup grated Parmesan cheese
- Salt and pepper to taste

Instructions

1. Preheat the oven to 375°F (190°C).
2. In a large bowl, combine the shredded chicken, cooked rice, condensed soup, milk, frozen vegetables, and Parmesan cheese. Season with salt and pepper.
3. Transfer the mixture to a greased baking dish.
4. Bake for 25-30 minutes, or until heated through and bubbly.

Baked Cod with Lemon and Herbs

Ingredients:
- 4 (4 oz) cod fillets
- 2 tablespoons olive oil
- 2 tablespoons lemon juice
- 1 teaspoon dried thyme
- 1 teaspoon dried parsley
- Salt and pepper to taste
- Lemon wedges for serving

Instructions
1. Preheat the oven to 400°F (200°C).
2. Place the cod fillets in a baking dish.

3. In a small bowl, whisk together the olive oil, lemon juice, thyme, parsley, salt, and pepper.
4. Pour the lemon and herb mixture over the cod fillets, ensuring they are evenly coated.
5. Bake for 15-20 minutes, or until the cod is cooked through and flakes easily with a fork.
6. Serve the baked cod with lemon wedges.

HEALTHY RECIPES

1. Avocado and Egg Toast Ingredients:
- 2 slices whole-grain bread
- 1 ripe avocado
- 2 eggs
- Salt and pepper to taste

Instructions
1. Toast the bread slices.
2. Mash the avocado and spread it evenly on the toasted bread.

3. Cook the eggs to your desired style (scrambled, sunny-side up, or poached).
4. Place the cooked eggs on top of the avocado toast.
5. Season with salt and pepper.

Quinoa and Vegetable Soup

Ingredients:

- 1 cup cooked quinoa
- 4 cups low-sodium vegetable or chicken broth
- 1 cup diced carrots
- 1 cup diced zucchini
- 1/2 cup diced celery
- Salt and pepper to taste
- Fresh herbs (e.g., parsley, dill) for garnish (optional)

Instructions

1. In a saucepan, bring the broth to a boil.
2. Add the carrots, zucchini, and celery. Reduce heat to medium-low and

simmer for 10-15 minutes, or until the vegetables are tender.

3. Stir in the cooked quinoa and season with salt and pepper to taste.
4. Garnish with fresh herbs if desired.

Baked Sweet Potato with Spinach and Feta

Ingredients:
- 2 medium sweet potatoes
- 2 cups fresh baby spinach
- 1/4 cup crumbled feta cheese
- 1 tablespoon olive oil
- Salt and pepper to taste

Instructions
1. Preheat the oven to 400°F (200°C).
2. Wash the sweet potatoes and prick them with a fork.
3. Bake the sweet potatoes for 45-60 minutes, or until tender when pierced with a fork.
4. In a skillet, sauté the spinach with olive oil until wilted.

5. Cut the baked sweet potatoes lengthwise and top with the sautéed spinach and crumbled feta cheese.
6. Season with salt and pepper.

Grilled Chicken Salad with Quinoa

Ingredients:
- 4 oz grilled chicken breast, sliced
- 1 cup cooked quinoa
- 2 cups mixed greens or baby spinach
- 1/2 cup sliced cucumber
- 1/4 cup sliced red bell pepper
- 2 tablespoons olive oil
- 2 tablespoons lemon juice or vinegar
- Salt and pepper to taste

Instructions
1. In a large bowl, combine the mixed greens or baby spinach, cooked quinoa, sliced cucumber, and sliced red bell pepper.
2. In a small bowl, whisk together the olive oil, lemon juice or vinegar, and salt and pepper to make a simple dressing.

3. Add the sliced grilled chicken to the salad and drizzle with the dressing.

Lentil and Vegetable Stew

Ingredients:
- 1 cup dried lentils, rinsed
- 4 cups low-sodium vegetable or chicken broth
- 1 cup diced carrots
- 1 cup diced zucchini
- 1 cup diced potatoes
- 1 teaspoon dried thyme
- Salt and pepper to taste

Instructions
1. In a large pot or Dutch oven, combine the lentils, broth, carrots, zucchini, potatoes, and thyme.
2. Bring the mixture to a boil, then reduce heat to low, cover, and simmer for 30-40 minutes, or until the lentils and vegetables are tender.
3. Season with salt and pepper to taste.

Deviled Eggs

Ingredients:

6 hard-boiled eggs

1/4 cup plain Greek yogurt

1 tablespoon Dijon mustard

1 tablespoon finely chopped fresh parsley (optional)

Salt and pepper to taste

Instructions:

Peel the hard-boiled eggs and cut them in half lengthwise.

Remove the yolks and place them in a bowl.

Mash the yolks with a fork.

Add the Greek yogurt, Dijon mustard, parsley (if using), and salt and pepper to taste. Mix well.

Spoon or pipe the yolk mixture back into the egg white halves.

Chill before serving.

Hummus and Vegetable Platter

Ingredients:

1 cup hummus

1 cup sliced cucumber

1 cup sliced bell peppers

1 cup carrot sticks

Whole-grain crackers or pita chips

Instructions:

Arrange the sliced cucumbers, bell peppers, and carrot sticks on a serving platter.

Place the hummus in a small bowl in the center of the platter.

Serve with whole-grain crackers or pita chips on the side.

Caprese Skewers

Ingredients:

1 pint cherry tomatoes

8 oz fresh mozzarella cheese, cut into small cubes

Fresh basil leaves

Balsamic glaze

Toothpicks

Instructions:

Thread a cherry tomato, a cube of mozzarella cheese, and a basil leaf onto a toothpick.

Repeat with the remaining ingredients.

Arrange the skewers on a serving platter.

Drizzle with balsamic glaze before serving.

Cucumber Bites

Ingredients:

1 English cucumber, sliced into rounds

1/2 cup cream cheese or plain Greek yogurt

1/4 cup finely chopped fresh dill or chives

Salt and pepper to taste

Instructions:

In a small bowl, mix the cream cheese or Greek yogurt with the chopped dill or chives. Season with salt and pepper.

Top each cucumber round with a small dollop of the cream cheese or yogurt mixture.

Chill before serving.

Avocado Boats

Ingredients:

2 ripe avocados

1/4 cup diced tomatoes

1/4 cup diced red onion

2 tablespoons fresh lime juice

Salt and pepper to taste

Instructions:

Cut the avocados in half lengthwise and remove the pits.

Scoop out a small amount of avocado flesh from each half to create a shallow well.

In a small bowl, mix the diced tomatoes, red onion, lime juice, and salt and pepper.

Spoon the tomato mixture into the avocado halves.

Chill before serving.

DESSERTS:

Baked Apples

Ingredients:

4 apples (such as Gala or Honeycrisp)

1/4 cup raisins or dried cranberries

1/4 cup chopped walnuts or pecans

2 tablespoons honey

1 teaspoon ground cinnamon

1/4 cup water

Instructions:

Preheat the oven to 375°F (190°C).

Core the apples, leaving the bottom intact.

In a small bowl, mix together the raisins or dried cranberries, chopped nuts, honey, and cinnamon.

Stuff the cored apples with the nut mixture.

Place the stuffed apples in a baking dish and pour the water into the bottom of the dish.

Bake for 30-40 minutes, or until the apples are tender when pierced with a fork.

Greek Yogurt Parfait

Ingredients:

1 cup plain Greek yogurt

1/2 cup fresh berries (such as strawberries, blueberries, or raspberries)

2 tablespoons honey or maple syrup

1/4 cup granola (low-fiber variety)

Instructions:

In a parfait glass or bowl, layer half of the Greek yogurt, followed by half of the berries and a drizzle of honey or maple syrup.

Repeat the layers with the remaining yogurt, berries, and honey or maple syrup.

Top with granola.

SNACKS:

Avocado Toast

 Ingredients:

2 slices whole-grain bread

1 ripe avocado

Lemon juice

Salt and pepper to taste

Instructions:

Toast the bread slices.

Mash the avocado with a fork and season with a squeeze of lemon juice, salt, and pepper.

Spread the mashed avocado evenly on the toasted bread.

Hummus and Veggie Sticks

Ingredients:

1 cup hummus

Assorted fresh veggies (such as carrots, cucumber, bell peppers, celery), cut into sticks

Instructions:

Arrange the veggie sticks on a plate or platter.

Place the hummus in a small bowl for dipping.

Trail Mix

Ingredients:

1/2 cup unsalted nuts (such as almonds, cashews, or pecans)

1/4 cup dried fruit (such as raisins, cranberries, or apricots)

2 tablespoons seeds (such as pumpkin or sunflower seeds)

Instructions:

In a bowl, mix together the nuts, dried fruit, and seeds.

Store the trail mix in an airtight container for up to a week.

"Congratulations on taking the first step towards a healthier, happier you! With the Quick and Easy Complete Solution Crohn's Disease Diet Cookbook for Seniors, you now have the tools and recipes to manage your Crohn's disease and enjoy delicious, nutritious meals that nourish your body and soothe your symptoms.

Remember, living with Crohn's disease doesn't mean you have to sacrifice flavor or convenience. With this cookbook, you can enjoy quick, easy, and gentle-on-the-stomach meals that support your health and well-being.

Don't let Crohn's disease hold you back any longer. Take control of your diet, your health, and your life. Cook with confidence, eat with joy, and live with freedom from the symptoms of Crohn's disease.

Happy cooking, and happy healing!"

This conclusion aims to:

- Congratulate the reader on taking the first step towards a healthier life
- Emphasize the benefits of the cookbook, including quick, easy, and nutritious meals
- Encourage the reader to take control of their health and well-being
- End with a positive and uplifting note, wishing the reader happy cooking and happy healing.

THE END

www.ingramcontent.com/pod-product-compliance
Lightning Source LLC
Chambersburg PA
CBHW071551260726
48653CB00007BA/2714